Drug Use and Evaluating Personality and Behavior Disorders

Problems Diagnosing Schizophrenia, Schizoaffective Disorder, and Bipolar

By: Lavoy Allison

Dedications

To: Selena for everything you do from saying my name to saying I love you. God bless you woman.

To: My family for living with me through the thick and thin of my schizophrenia and loving me when I was at my worse. That love meant so much in my recovery.

To: My readers for looking into this book and understanding either your mental illness more or your family or friend's illness better. If you want to read my other books you can search my name Lavoy Allison at Amazon!

Table of Contents

Chapter 1: What Defines Schizophrenia?

I was first diagnosed with Schizophrenia in 2002. Today is 2019 and I am just now getting the hang of having the illness. It is not like the cold where you get the illness once and you remember the symptoms. This illness is the freakiest of all. Do you think you can get shot at and it not hurt you? How about drive into another car and your car not get damaged? It seems cool to you while the illness is in full affect but when you come down you realize what you were thinking and could have done. It scared the straight up hell out of me. Those are just some of the delusions of Schizophrenia.

When I was diagnosed did I have the illness of schizophrenia? No I didn't, I had gotten through the worse part. I had medicated with cannabis on the streets to get better. What did the doctor do? Give me a medicine like outdated Prozac to bring back the symptoms I had because I caught him feeling up a mentally ill female that would walk nude through the halls of the wing we were on in the mental hospital. When I reported him, he made my life a mental hell again.

Have you heard voices telling you that a loved one died? I did. I heard one tell me that Selena flat-lined and I prayed to God that I wanted to die and didn't even think to pray for her to be okay. I prayed that the Lord would understand I was tired and couldn't give love another chance. I prayed that God would find me some bad people to harass and have dirty cops show up so I could die serving my country as I once thought that I might.

While I didn't find anyone to kill or kill me that night, I smelt gun powder. The cops tried to shoot me and the gun miss fired. I haven't done much thinking about how lucky I am. I have just been thinking about how cool our Lord is for letting me and Selena live. Currently I am still in a treatment facility but at least I know I will be okay and have a chance at a life with Selena. That keeps me going despite the illness I now have.

I have depression and because I said that I work for the CIA I am 'schizophrenic.' As for the CIA they left me here to cool off. I took it on myself to take the education they gave me to prepare a report on the state of the current mental health treatment I am getting. When I got poisoned I ate a lot of cannabis and smoked a lot to so I got better. It treats schizophrenia better and faster than any pill I have ever used.

At times my schizophrenia had lead me to believe that I was in control of the planet and it was my job to clean it up. Also I believed I was here to witness and judge for the Lord. It was a time when I didn't have any love in my heart. I had gotten poisoned and believed I was God. I had to learn to read, write, and talk again while not knowing any of my past. At the same time I had to fight Satan. I was feeling things like the nails Jesus felt and the crown of thorns. I didn't believe in learning about hell or bad things but I got a crash course in it. That was the effects of the poisons I was exposed to.

At that time I believed that I was having to go through these things to help the Lord design hell for really bad people. I admit it now. I was off my rocker but I didn't think anything about it. I believed I was chosen by God to help create where he will send people the lake of fire. Yes I thought I was designing hell. And if you haven't repented you damn sure better now! God will go easy on cussing if you understand that religion wars is those following the beast and the Lord just wants you to believe, do right, help yourself, others, the animals and the planet. Planting a tree once and a while won't hurt either. Religion has started war after war and more people have died because of religion. If someone believes the Lord is God and that is whom they obey and follow in the teachings of the laws they are right before God.

So do you think I am crazy, I didn't then but I am glad I got medical cannabis to get past that. I had to do that on my own by the way. I look back and see I was in a delusion. I know that it isn't politically correct anymore to say crazy but there again I haven't seen that society has changed much from those terms. I have been called a fuckin loon and other names too. The best thing to do is as the good Lord says. It is only words and they will hurt the person speaking such in hell. But while you see that someone is cussing you for things you did or do while in a crisis of mental illness remember God wants you to do right. Maybe those harsh words are the Devil tempting you. Remember talking bad things about someone will bring bad things. Even if it is in hell they go through what you did with your illness. Maybe for eternity at that.

While Schizophrenia is a big word always remember that our Lord is bigger. If you have ever wondered about where they got the idea for the staff and snakes for the medical insignia I will tell you. The staff is your faith in God and the two snakes are the devil and Satan attacking your faith. The wings in it are the angels that study medicine that try to help you along. You can't leave the Lord out of the recovery from your illness. Remember that too. That is the strongest help I think I can give you.

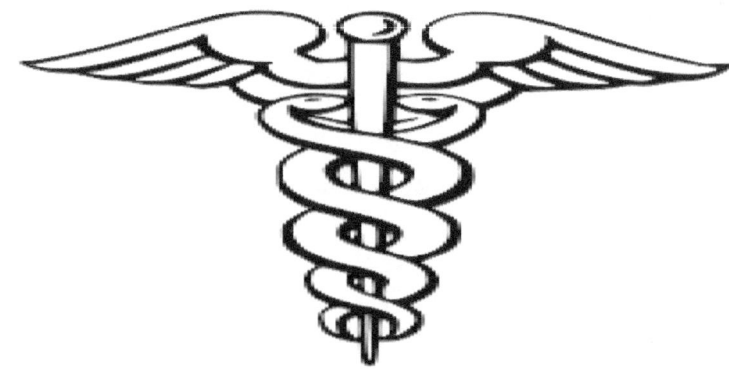

Schizophrenia defined is hard to understand without an example as I went through. You have the five hallucinations and false beliefs also known as delusions all together and that defines schizophrenia. End of chapter right? I think not!?! I would like you to know that mental health treatment is getting better but only slowly. The doctors as of 2020 are still not prescribing medical cannabis in mental hospitals. I was in the mental hospital in 2002 and they didn't really teach you how to know when you are having a relapse as they do today. In 2002 I was just told what my illness was and was given different medicines. And trust me they tried me on many different pills to get it right. I felt like a lab rat but today I am glad I went through it to some point. I have my life back and I helped make some changes to the mental health treatment plans.

 I said symptoms of schizophrenia has the five hallucinations. Do you know them? Unfortunately I do because of going through them and recently have to learn them. I must say I thought many people were lying when they said they were sick and hearing voices before I went through it. Also I asked them if they were smoking weed sprayed with embalming fluid and they said no. Why didn't I just believe them in 1995? Because I started smoking cannabis that wasn't poisoned so I wasn't hearing voices and others were getting poisoned. They would say that they started hearing voices when they started smoking weed. I thought they were lying to keep from working. When it happened to me I was a believer. I heard voices, seen things that weren't there, smelt things that weren't there, felt things that weren't there, and I would taste things that weren't there. All five of the hallucinations.

 Now we are getting into the crazy of the crazy right? Yeah you can taste and smell things that are not there. Most of us have heard of hearing and seeing things and possibly feeling things but I bet I got you with the smelling and tasting things right!?! Remember if you smoke cannabis and start hearing voices it is not the cannabis. There is something in it that someone laced it with. Any drug that is a medicine can be abused though. Remember to talk to a doctor about your use but understand not all doctors are on the same page with the poisons being the problem.

Next, to be schizophrenic you must have the hallucinations and the false beliefs too. So you can have Grandiose delusions(false beliefs) that you are someone famous when you are not or Erotomanic which is the belief that you are married to a celebrity and they are in love with you when that is not true. Other delusions are jealous, persecutory, somatic, and mixed. With schizophrenia you can have one or more of these delusions and you will not know the difference from them and reality.

Chapter 2: Schizophrenia and Treatment

So I guess we need to get into treatment of schizophrenia. Let's start by saying I have been treated for 17 years and if I was to get off my medicine the doctor prescribed I would relapse and the symptoms would come back. Please do take note that I have not been treated by a doctor with cannabis. Only pharmaceutical pills that are trial and error. I have found some prescription pills that work since then though. The treatment facility I am in will not allow me to use cannabis. I now take Abilify 30 mg and Lexipro 20 mg once daily. I deal with the side affects of weight gain and constipation. Luckily I went through enough cannabis to get past the worst part. If you have ever seen a schizophrenic person in a mental hospital you would understand the illness better. If they would treat them with cannabis they would come back around faster and be 'reachable.'

The main thing that I have noticed is that I don't get severe depression near as much now that I am taking the Abilify and the Lexipro together. I am doing much better. I still see flashes of light and get depressed some. I have been on the Lexipro and Abilify together since January 2017 and it is now June 2019. I spent my time reading my Bible and studying self help books to learn more about developing websites and server administration. I also learn about programming some. I spent some time doing matrix math problems also so that I could get my brain going again. I still do all these things too. I believe studying and relearning is part of the cure.

Why would I mention studying math and computer science as part of the cure? Because the brain is just like a muscle or joint in the body. It needs exercise to get better. You can do three sheets of math or about one hundred math problems and then read a book and your outlook on life and your health will change I promise you it will. I know from experience and my letters to the government has caused classes to be taught in mental health hospitals. They don't teach you math and reading but they have classes now. Mental hospitals now have to teach people about their mental illness and coping skills. Either way you have to get your brain going again.

What do you mean by getting your brain going again you ask? I got some bad weed and before I tried to get myself killed by the cops I was seeing things and hearing things. I found out that reading writing and math helps get the bad chemicals out of the brain and your mind back to normal. But the catch is that you have to want it. If you know schizophrenia or someone that has it the worst part is they like the company of the voices sometimes and do not want them to leave. You have to interact with them or you yourself has to interact with others to see the light as they say. Anyway I had the delusions again that I was here to judge the end of sin on earth for the Lord the last time I got poisoned. I was seeing flashes of light and Godzilla in a fourth dimension.

Yes I believed I was seeing into another dimension and

was seeing Godzilla do the work for God by forcing the bad people to clean the streets and getting the dead bodies and things out of the waterways. The people the bad guys hurt or took family away from they had to go through hell in front of them. Okay yes I believe it would help people believe God is a cool motherfucker (and he is) if the sinners fixed the planet and made it easier for the believers. Tell Lord God your ideas I think he is open for some new ways to punish and reward.

Back on track that was what was going through my mind. I got arrested and the doctor put me on something that made me even worse. I was telling my attorney that the pale horse the Bible talks about in the book of Revelations was one of the creatures in the Aliens movie and that they meant pale green. I was in the butt naked cell for three months. It was bad. I finally made it out and got the address to Washington and the C.I.A. office. One thing about working for the government you still technically are not suppose to break the law. I did anyway. Why? Because I talk about being poisoned and it keeping from them legalizing cannabis and people start poisoning me. I found one of the drug dealers supplying bad weed and I went wild crazy on him.

I told you that I prayed to find bad people and draw out bad cops. I didn't tell you that I had done dumb crap like this before for the government. When I said that the mental health hospitals were getting better I wasn't kidding. I have been on the case since 2002! If you want to know the truth I am partly responsible for the mental illness training classes you have to take.

I am not saying that the state mental hospitals have it

all right. I am just saying they better prepare you for life with your illness. I think they need to remind mentally ill people that learning math and reading teach multi-tasking and it is important in the treatment of an illness. It has greatly helped me!

If for say you end up in a mental health hospital don't play around and not try to learn how to take care of yourself and prevent a mental illness relapse. You will get stuck in the system and now you have to be on voluntary status to get out! What is that about you ask? You have to pass the mental doctor's evaluation before you can get out. Why? Because they are trying to save your lives and keep you from making decisions like I did that got me shot at and arrested.

To start treatment the doctor will give you an assessment which will be a list of questions they ask you. Have you ever heard voices? Have you ever used drugs and what are the drugs you used? Have you seen things that no one else could see? Questions like that are what they will ask. Just be honest and try not to get scared. It is important for them to know the truth so they can properly diagnosis you. That way they will not get the idea that you need a medicine that you don't. Some of the medicines will make you worse causing other symptoms and that you do not want.

When they decide that you have schizophrenia they will prescribe you something and suggest treatment like counseling. If you do not wish to be hospitalized and you do not seem like you will hurt yourself or others you can go home. If you are in a delusion and out to kill yourself or someone you will be best hospitalized for a while. Don't worry it happens to the best of us.

One of the classes you will have when you have a mental illness like schizophrenia is Illness Management and Recovery. In that class you will learn to set personal goals and make progress to recovery. You will learn about mental illness and the process to recover. In learning so you will learn to decrease symptoms and reduce relapse as well as time having to be in a hospital.

Of these steps you will always want to start with setting your goals because you need something to work toward. While you may have symptoms longer than you like if you have goals that you can reach while in treatment you will find hope in reaching a goal. That seems like a baby step to some but it is a lunar step for many. There are some people that are stuck in their delusions and they need those 'small steps.' Some are in severe crisis and depression and need those goals for the hope they bring. Remember that means a lot to some. And never look at those small steps as a disgrace. Don't look down on people either. While many are victims of poisoned drugs they deserve a safe nonjudgmental environment to recover in.

Maybe recovery for you isn't such a short term goal you just want the voices to stop. The focus then would be to develop your own recovery process and plan. Doctors know that no two cases of mental illness are the same but you must take part in recovery and sometimes that is recovery as a group. Therapy is going to help more than you know. Once you sit in a group and see that others are having the same problems it will be a little easier to talk to someone or the group.

I remember when it seem that I was the only one that would understand my problems and no one else would. It made me even worse. Sometimes you have to listen in a group setting to understand how to address your illness. That was part of my problem. I didn't know the medical terms to discuss with a doctor. What I was going through was too hard for me to explain.

Some of the skills you will learn is why not to mix drugs and alcohol into your recovery plan. Remember please that these studies are based on medical ways before the legalization of cannabis for medical use and there is no study on it in many states. I now live in Florida and they just legalized cannabis for medical use in 2016. It is June 2019 and there has been no change in the medical teachings and some doctors are still stressing that cannabis is an abused drug and not talking about it as a good medicine. They haven't switched to talking about what the poisoned drugs are doing and focusing on the poisons either. That is where the doctors making the medicine are getting it wrong. Some think this is intentional.

While cannabis can be over used it is a medicine and one that many of our pills are made from. That is something that other countries do not want the government of the United States to understand or let be known to the public. Also the side effects we have are from the chemicals they use to keep the pills from getting you high like cannabis.

Part of recovery and coping is learning to deal with the voices and hallucinations while they are happening. There are many ways to deal you just have to know what works for you. I listen to music, surf the internet, read, write, and study to get my mind off things like the voices and the things I see. You may have other ways to get your self to a better way of thinking and forget about the things that are happening in your mind.

There is also meditating and muscle relaxation techniques that will help you. I have seen people exercise and sing to the music playing. You will want to make sure that you learn some of these techniques so that you can see the light at the end of the tunnel. Also you don't want to let your illness take you over. When you start to hear voices or see things start your relaxation techniques and coping skills to stop yourself from thinking about them before depression sets in and you are having a full blown relapse.

Chapter 3: What Defines Schizoaffective Disorder

So what defines Schizoaffective disorder? Well that will include a number of things. Schizoaffective Disorder is a combination of Schizophrenia and Bipolar Disorders. With Schizoaffective Disorder you will have a combination of delusions, hallucinations, and mood extremes like depression or mania. I was once labeled Schizoaffective Depressed type.

As I said before the delusions are false beliefs that people hold even when there is evidence against the belief. Sadly it can be as simple as believing that someone is following them or that song lyrics are their own. Some delusional people hold the belief that people are talking to them in songs. Sometimes yet rarely it is possible to get misdiagnosed because you can not prove your story so be careful and carry proper identification.

Doctors look for sudden changes in your personality and go from there. Have you been happy for weeks and then crash for weeks and not know why? You have a symptom. Do you suffer from confusion and possible delirium? You have symptoms of Schizoaffective Disorder. One of the things a doctor will evaluate is if you can or can not focus.

When do you want to see a doctor with these symptoms you ask? As soon as possible. Remember that your brain is becoming chemically unstable and you are not you. Anything could happen! You want to first let your family and/or loved ones know what is happening with you. The best thing is to be honest. It could mean life or death if you get around the wrong people. Sometimes people do not understand mental illness and react to soon. I tried to get shot by the police because I didn't think the bullets would hit me and I about got shot. I smelt gun powder. I was unarmed and at the time I smelt gun powder I had my hands on top of my head for five minutes to show I was not a danger. I was cussing them and talking about their drug connection but anyway.

What are the warning signs you ask? When symptoms appear quickly without reason. If you suddenly get depressed without reason you need to seek help. There is no reason to soak in your sorrow and it take on other symptoms that may lead you to hurt yourself or someone else. If you believe you are going to hurt yourself or others it is time to seek help for yourself or have a family member seek help for you. Also remember you could have had a head injury that may have lead to your illness and the doctor will check for this. Most of the time it is a safe experience in the evaluation.

During the physical exam that comes with the mental exam you will be checked for fever, a rapid heart beat, confusion, and things that might not be right with your brain usually through and MRI at times. Needless to say your physical health has a lot to do with your mental state. You want to remember to eat regularly and get enough sleep. Eating and sleeping or the lack there of are also signs that you are not feeling well and need to see the doctor.

I mentioned that delusions and hallucinations are a part of Schizoaffective Disorder but there is also the mood extremes. You will have either mania or depression. Mania is where you are in a state of high all the time. I was told that mania was much like the symptoms of ADHD. Depression is what most of us understand the most because everyone has been sad at one time or the other. What makes these symptoms a medical issue is when the mood extremes last for unusually long amounts of time.

Okay so what can you do if you are not getting better fast enough? Get a Medical Cannabis card. Only buy from an approved dispensary. That way you don't get poisoned through street weed and get worse. Focus on medicating with eatables at first. You can smoke to medicate but you need to focus on getting your cannabis sugar (the medicine) levels up. Some pills they treat mental illnesses with require blood work to see how high the levels (the amount of medicine) is in your blood. Some of the blood work is to see how hard you body is taking the chemicals they use in the medicine. Some of those meds cause liver and kidney failure.

Chapter 4: What Defines Bipolar Disorder

When you get into what defines Bipolar you are talking about the two extremes of Mood. To be diagnosed Bipolar you have to carry one of the moods for around a week to two weeks and then go to the other extreme within a days time and have it for a week to two weeks. Simply put you have extreme moods often and for long periods of time.

You will have these symptoms of extreme moods that appear suddenly and without warning. One of the first things that the doctor is going to try to do is get you on medicine that will help level out your moods to where you seem 'normal.' These mood extremes can include rage and no expression of emotion. If you have not had these then you may never understand completely because many times unless someone has been diagnosed you may never catch it because these illnesses happen to normal people and some carry it well.

At one time I was labeled with having Bipolar Schizoaffective Disorder. I carried that for sometime. I have slowly gotten better but I am still diagnosed as having Schizophrenia. I didn't have proper identification and was claiming my government job when I was arrested. I even tried to get the doctor I had to see to call the CIA office for me. I was seen as mentally unstable and put in the butt naked cell. It didn't help I was trying to bust another cop cartel.

I will have to get reevaluated when I get in touch with headquarters. I was poisoned and had to take medicine that made me worse when I reported a doctor for illegal activity. I have worked hard to get better with the medicine I am on. The math, reading and prayer helped more than anything. Finally I got a doctor that realized that I could be telling the truth about working for the government. A good point to remember is to keep your nose clean and remember your service number! Please remember not to lie or get angry during your health care because it could falsely look like another symptom. If you feel they are not treating you right get a second opinion. That is your right as long as you do it respectfully.

Sometimes you will not be able to notice your own relapse so it is a good thing to journal your daily activities and thoughts so you can see what you are thinking on paper. Also use your coping skills and remember them like the back of your hand.

Chapter 5: Friends or Foes

I am sure that you have heard the phrase that your friends are only friends when you have money to spend on them. Sometimes telling your friends you have a mental illness is not going to go over to well. Especially if you have an episode in front of them. Family can be the same way. If someone does not understand about the illness then they can really hurt your feelings. If you can keep from hurting someone that has a mental illness.

My mom and dad hurt my feelings bad. I was hearing voices and seeing things. I was feeling things too. They told me to quit doing drugs so I could go back to work and help out with the bills. I had gotten poisoned. Needless to say if you have been through lack of remorse from loved ones about your symptoms then you know. It was like they didn't care what I was going through or that I needed help, they were worried about the money. I wasn't raised where you go to the doctor at least twice a year I had no idea what to do. I just knew that smoking cannabis made the voices stop and made me feel better. It even helped me sleep.

With me not knowing anything about modern medicine I thought I was doing the right thing. The only problem was that I was cut off from pure cannabis and the cops were having everyone around me that sold cannabis deal their poisoned weed. Tobacco insecticide, embalming fluid, anti-freeze, battery acid and strict-nine. I was just getting sicker and the schizophrenia was getting worse.

That is what happens when you stand up to a cop cartel and try to keep their kids from raping women and running wild but anyway.

The friends I thought I had were the enemy and they made my life hell. You could be in a similar situation. I reported to Washington that these poisons are the problem and I was right. Many people over the last couple of decades have been poisoned through the drugs they used. That is why your parents and everyone tell you to stay off drugs. It isn't just medicine anymore. they have poisoned a lot of the medicine on the streets and call it drugs.

If you are not getting your cannabis from a dispensary or growing your own organically then you are at a high risk for an illness. Don't take the risk I am telling you from experience that schizophrenia is not worth a few good highs if you are lucky enough to get a few highs before getting the illness. Besides you can get cancer along with those voices from those poisons they put in street drugs.

Basically I am saying that a drug dealer is not always the best person to make your friend. Your 'friend' may damn well be the foe that takes you to the grave. They are poisoning the cannabis before it comes into this country. People are putting tobacco insecticide on cannabis because they found that it has embalming fluid in it.

You don't have to spray outdoor cannabis for bugs. You can spray the ground around. The plant I grew outside didn't get touched by anything that would eat on it and I didn't even spray around it. Why then do they put it on there? To make it more of a high they say but there is fact that it kills the effects of the THC and the poisons just mess with your head. It can make you really dead too. Ever heard of K2 killing people. That is what they are using on it. Just smelling embalming fluid can cause brain and lung cancer. Just think about inhaling it?

So are these suicidal people that are selling these poisons your friends or trying to take people with them when they die? I think you need to buy some cannabis seeds from the seed bank and grow your own if you are just going to do it anyway. Like I said talk to your parents or family and make a safety net. It might save your life. Besides they could be cool about it and let you use cannabis at home. Why? Because they love you and at least if you do it at home they don't have to worry about you not making it home!

While you are out to see who your friends are and are not, remember that through it all you should be able to trust in your doctor. I have had problems with doctors because I reported them and still had to see them. This should not happen on a wide scale basis but remember it can occur that you get a bad doctor. Find a new one as quick as you can. Remember that you need the treatment and you need to get better. Also remember that doctors before legalization were not allowed to prescribe cannabis or tell you to use. They are not at fault.

Chapter 6: Medicines Cause Side Affects. You Want Me to Take It Too?

Many if not all of the medicines that doctors will give you will have side affects. Yes that is part of the problem. Many people do not get that instant cure like with cannabis and the doctors have made most of their money from the prescriptions they write. Huh, you say? Yes the pharmaceutical companies were giving doctors a percentage of what they make from the pill sales. I wrote President George Bush Jr. and he put in motion a law against it. That is what we have to do and if you know of anything wrong with <u>anything</u> write your government officials.

I was given the assignment when I enlisted to do what I could to study and see if there was a way to legalize some of the street drugs. The government knows that it is costing them to much for having them illegal. I went and prayed to God and cannabis was the first and only drug so far that I have helped get legalized. God put medicines on the planet to cure us. He wants us well but some people have stood in the way of that. It is getting better slowly

You didn't know that the government is trying to see the other side of the story did you? Yes the government is wanting to get some of the drugs on the street that are used as medicines legalized so the killing and stealing will quit. There are government officials that do care about the people in the United States and love you too. Those are the ones that have God in their hearts and pray for us all. But with the poisoning of cannabis they are slow to legalize it straight out or any other drug for that matter.

The government is also doing what they can to get our medicines to have lesser or no side effects so that they are safer. You have to remember that we as citizens need to help the government fix these problems too. If you get a bad drug tell someone. Write the Surgeon General's office and the President. They don't take all the medicines that are on the shelves so do your part and tell someone.

Remember that these pharmaceutical drugs are made from things like cannabis so yes the government wants the legalization of it to stop other types of poisoning and drug addictions. I just want you to know that things like this take time and you need to know the full truth before you vote. Many prescription drugs are made from cannabis, cocaine, efedrin, and opium that are being imported from fields that are being sprayed with insecticides like DDT! Many of you do not know this. These insecticides are what cause the side effects.

They even use chemicals that keep the medicines from getting you high. God knew what he was doing when he made these medicines and the getting high part can treat depression. Ask someone about to commit suicide to smoke a blunt first and if it is good medical cannabis they will change their mind 99% of the time.

You now know about people using street drugs and have seen what happens when people used poisoned drugs. Some people go further than I did. They kill people and steal while trying not to work. Vote wisely please and remember medicine from cannabis or any of these other medicines called drugs will be cheaper not coming from the pharmaceutical companies. The government is looking for the cheapest way that the side effects will not be as bad. One answer is coming from companies following Food and Drug Administration (FDA) rules like the medical cannabis dispensaries.

Thank you for reading my book and taking a look into the truth about Personality and Behavior Disorders. Please do not take for granite what I have told you about prescription medicines and the legalization of cannabis and other medicines sold as drugs. Bless you all and remember to keep the Lord in your heart during any illness!

Also remember that the best treatment for COVID-19 is the ingredient they use in Meth, efedrin. You can get it in sudofedrin cold pills. I had pneumonia and malaria at different times and Speed Pills also known as White Crosses treated them well. Speed sold as Heads Up pills in 1994 in purer form than sudofedrin is what I used to treat myself for my respiratory illnesses. I am working to get the government to study this cure. Sadly when they outlawed Heads Up and other White Cross speed products they may not have a good supply and that is the reason for the cautions taken.